LOW BACK PAIN

A FRANK Look at Natural Back Pain Relief

by

Frank Gresham CMTPT

© Frank Gresham 2013

What's a **FRANK** Book?

Finally
Real
Advice
'**N**'
Know-how

To Get Rid of
Your Pain
Naturally!

Is it an adventure to get in and out of a chair?

Does it hurt to get out of bed?

Is it hard to pick up your child or grandchild?

Did you have to stop enjoying sports?

Here's a novel idea:

Stop masking your pain with drugs.

Discover WHY you have low back pain and correct it!

Learn the real causes and perpetuating factors of pain in your lower back. Get rid of them and start feeling better!

Important Legal Stuff

Dedication

This book is dedicated to George S. Pellegrino

He taught me that I can be me when I'm with my patients. Laughter with knowledge works wonders together.

We need to laugh at ourselves sometimes, and George, you taught me that. You are truly missed my friend. God bless you and your family.

Acknowledgements

First and foremost, I want to give praise to Jesus Christ. He has allowed me to be pain free and blessed me with the ability to help others with their pain. He is, after all, the Great Physician.

I want to acknowledge the love of my life, Deborah Ann Gresham. I strongly believe in God because of the angel he placed by my side for over 34 years. Without her love and support I would not be the man that I am today. I am on bended knee when I say, "Thank you, my Beautiful Bride."

Thank you to Nancy Shaw for teaching me about Dr.Janet Travell's protocol and her wisdom on "WHY" we hurt.

My mother, for helping me get started with my practice.

George and Vicky at AIMS (American Institute of Myofascial Studies.) Your friendship and school has enabled me to achieve my dreams. I will be forever grateful

A special thank you to Kathryn Merrow. Her dedication and hunger for getting this word out to the rest of the world is inspiring. Thank you for our new found friendship

Table of Contents

Introduction

I discovered Frank in a pain relief forum online and I could tell right off the bat that he knew what he was talking about.

Frank has a unique understanding of how bodies work. He knows why pain happens and what to do to prevent or stop it. It was my pleasure to interview Frank for you.

And, I know you will enjoy his helpful videos about self-treatment for lower back pain. The links to the videos are included in this book.

– Kathryn Merrow, The Pain Relief Coach

Why natural pain relief?

Kathryn: How did you get interested in the field of natural pain relief, Frank?

Frank: Well, it started for me quite a few years ago. I had chronic back pain and migraines for probably 25 years and I was first told it was allergies. I was given a mild pain pill to help me with my pain but since I was unknowingly still doing the same things that were causing my pain, it kept getting worse and worse.

During the last four or five years of this painful time in my life, I was on a lot of pain medication. And I was always searching; I was doing yoga, I was stretching, I had a hot tub.

I was trying to do anything I could think of to ease the pain with no success.

Then one day, about eleven or twelve years ago, a chiropractor friend of mine told me, 'You need to go see this person who does trigger point therapy'. Never heard of it before and I thought, 'You know what, I tried everything else. I'll try.'

Well, the first time I saw this therapist, I could tell that she knew what my problem was. She showed me my pain patterns on a chart, she checked my hip height, and we talked about sleep positions for me.

I slept on my back which was a good position, but I had my arms over my head when I slept. When I stopped putting my arms over my head, it took the stress out of the trapezius (upper back) muscles and the SCM (sternocleidomastoid) muscles in my neck. Those muscles were able to relax and I could tell a difference within the first week of doing this.

And when I was getting the treatment work done, a light bulb just went on for me. I thought, 'This is so awesome and I know people don't know about this because I never heard about it myself.' I just had to learn it; I had no more headaches!

And from the second visit on, I just remember saying, 'How do I do this? Do you have to go to school for years?' And thank goodness you didn't so I was able to study anatomy and physiology and actually go to a school that taught all the principles and practices of trigger point therapy and pain patterns.

I've just been fascinated with it ever since and I've been trying to pass it on to other folks. I feel I've been blessed to be pain free now and I enjoy helping others achieve that same goal.

The most common causes of low back pain

Kathryn: Frank, let's talk about low back pain. Why do people have pain in their lower backs? What do you do to help them when they come to see you?

Frank: Well, when a new patient comes into my office, I usually find there are a couple of reasons why they have problems with low back pain.

A lot of times, it's their sleep position as well as lack of proper stretches for their pain.

A lot of folks sleep on their stomach or they use a half side/half stomach sleep position. These are very, very bad positions for the muscles. They are bad positions for back pain. If you are sleeping twisted up all night, how can you expect to stand up straight the next morning?

Stomach sleeping is probably the worst position, or one of the worst positions for you to sleep in because it stretches out the front of the body, the abdominal muscles, and shortens the back muscles. You must sleep in a neutral posture that doesn't put tension into the muscles. You can get back pain and also headaches, vertigo, shoulder and neck pain and more when sleeping on your stomach.

Once you change your sleeping position to a more neutral side or back position you will reduce the tension in your muscles.

The other sleep position that causes lower back pain is when people sleep on their side in the fetal position. Folks will sleep with one leg rolled over in front of the other, and that's straining their hip all night, so I show them a more neutral position so the muscles will be relaxed in the morning. I always try to have them sleep with their ear, shoulder and hip in alignment.

You want your muscles to be relaxed while you sleep so they will be relaxed when you wake up. Once you correct your sleep position you won't be in so much pain when you wake up. You will actually be refreshed after making these changes.

Kathryn: So, a lot of people think sleeping in the fetal position is the ideal position to be in but you're telling me no?

Frank: Exactly. The stomach muscle that refers to low back pain is the rectus abdominis. It attaches to the pubic bone and up into the ribs.

When the rectus abdominis muscle is shortened, there are two main pain referral patterns.

1. The first is across the low back, from side to side in the waistline area.

2. The other one's up higher and goes across the bra line and people get pain up there too when that muscle's short.

This is common with a low back patient. I had a new patient last week and even though I hadn't even worked on him yet I asked him to change his sleep position. I also gave him a heel lift to level out his hips and his pain was gone by 70% or 80% when I saw him three days later.

Kathryn: Very interesting.

Other possible causes for low back pain

Kathryn: Are there some other possible causes for low back pain.

Frank: Yes, absolutely! We will talk about them, too.

One of the very first things I do for a patient when they come in for a consult is to make sure they're comfortable. A lot of times when people have back pain, they keep moving around in the chair because they can't get comfortable. They are off balance and that can come from uneven hip heights.

Once I find out which side of their body is lower as they are sitting, I have them sit in a chair on an ischial lift (a pad that is placed under one 'sit' bone, often about 3/8 of an inch thick) all of a sudden you can just see them relax and go, 'this feels good'. Their body senses it and that makes a big difference because the muscles are relaxing so the person is finally able to relax. The muscles are not working against each another.

So, we start off with three things to check and do:

1. First, if you have a short leg, we use a heel lift to make sure your hips are level when you are standing.

2. Second, we also have to make sure that your hips are leveled when you are sitting, so we put an ischial lift under the ischium when you sit. The ischium is also called the 'sit bone.'

3. The third thing that we check for is Morton's Toe.

The toe that causes low back pain

Another cause and perpetuating factor for low back pain is Morton's Toe.

Morton's Toe is when the second toe or the second metatarsal bone's a little longer than the big toe, and you're actually walking on an ice skate blade when you have Morton's Toe. That causes muscle dysfunction as you're walking. You're walking on the ice skate blade instead of a tripod (three parts of your foot) as you should.

You should carry your weight from your heel to your big toe and little toe, so you're connecting all three points. If you have Morton's Toe you're wavering back and forth in your shoe and that's causing strain on your calf muscles and your thigh muscles, and it can transfer all the way up to cause lower back pain.

I've had folks start to feel better within days after I put the little insert in their shoes for Morton's Toe. Often patients can tell something feels better almost instantly once they have the insert in their shoe. They're all, 'Hey! This is different.' They can feel it. They can sense it.

Kathryn: How many people have this Morton's Toe structure?

Frank: I would say about 75% whether they know it or not. I'm really surprised at how many people have it but here's a really easy way to tell if you do: Look down. Is your second toe longer than your big toe?

Also, if you check on the outside of your big toe there's usually a callus. Sometimes it's very faint and other times its so bad that people will sand it down or go get a pedicure or something to that effect to make it smooth.

The callus is caused by your foot moving back and forth in your shoe, and that brings up another point: shoes play an important role in back pain. You've got to have the shoe that fits you correctly; if the shoe is too tight and you have Morton's Toe, it's a double whammy.

Kathryn: So, there are many potential things that could be causing back pain, but you do something different than most when people come to you.

What do you do to help people?

Frank: Well, I follow Dr. Janet Travell's protocol. She was President Kennedy's White House physician. She's the doctor that got him pretty much free of his back pain. She has a protocol that I follow and with that protocol, I'm finding why you have back pain and not just treating the site of the pain.

Steps to Determine Whether You Need a Correction or Posture corrective Insole:

1) When I see that someone has Morton's Toe, I explain to them that they are walking on the blade of an ice skate, basically, and that's why they pronate (drop their arch) which can give them knee pain or low back pain just to name a few. Once the correction is put in their shoe, they will then walk on all three points of their foot correctly. They will be more sturdy and balanced. No more "weak ankles."

2) The insert fits into the patient's shoes. It's a full insert with a raised area (that starts at 3.5 mm in height) under the big toe. This allows the big toe to make contact with the surface first and totally takes the more dominant toe (the second, longer toe) out of the picture when the body decides how to walk.

Please go to the home page on my website http://TheChronicPainCenter.com to see how to order these inserts. Just click on the symbol of the two shoes at the bottom of that page.

3) The inserts in your shoes allow your foot to function correctly. Without the inserts all the muscles in the feet, legs, hips have been working in a dysfunctional manner because of the pronation. Most patients notice a difference immediately. It's like getting a front end alignment on your car. If you have new tires you want them the same size— they need to be balanced and aligned properly. If you don't do that, they will wear down quickly and most likely vibrate when driving the car. The same can be said about our feet and the shoes we wear. Many folks require a heel lift to balance out the hips and take stress off the rest of the body.   Then we need to align the feet to make sure they don't put any undue pressure on the ankle, knee or any other body parts. Once this is done the car--and the body--are balanced and aligned thus eliminating stress on the joints and muscles.

So, the first things I want to find out are, 'Okay, are your hips uneven? Do you have Morton's toe? Do you sleep in a bad position? Do you take in too much sugar during the day?'

Sugar's a big deal, especially in our country where we just eat too much of it, so that's something else we have to look at.

I can think of two or three patients right off the top of my head; one gentleman in particular had a bad shoulder pain. He was drinking four carbonated sodas a day and I said, 'You know what? Before I can even work on you to correct anything else, the hip height and such, you have to stop drinking the cola because that's contributing to your pain.' And he was a little upset because he had to give that up.

He came back into my office maybe 7 or 10 days later. He's touching his shoulder where it hurt and he says, 'This is 80%, 90% gone. It's just very faint and you haven't even worked on me yet.'

I know it was the sugar. There are 11 teaspoons of sugar in a soda, so he was having like 45 to 50 teaspoons of sugar a day. That was suppressing his immune system. It was not allowing his body to heal and it was also hyper-irritating the muscles.

When people get off sugar, they notice a difference in their pain. And diet sweeteners are no better!

Kathryn: When you say sugar, you mean any of the sweeteners that are not low calorie, right?

Frank: Correct. Also, I know somebody who says, 'Well, orange juice is good for you and I drink a quart of orange juice a day.' Actually, that's too much orange juice. If you typically sit down and eat an orange, you might have one, maybe two at the most, but when you drink too much sugar, even if it's natural sugar, it's still too much for the body.

You have to do things in moderation.

I don't want people to think, 'Oh no, I can't have chocolate cake ever again,' or, 'I can't have a treat,' or any kind of sweets. Yes, you can. Everything should be in moderation. My patients have to be free of sugar before I can work on them. After they are out of pain and doing well, they can have sweets again. But, only in moderation. That means very small amounts.

Remember, too much sugar irritates the muscles--so be sensible!

Kathryn: Will you please tell us about trigger points? Please explain them.

Frank: Well, your muscles have memory. When I explain that to people, I usually ask them, 'What did you like to do when you were more active? Did you play a sport?'

Sometimes people will say they played golf or tennis so let's say it's golf. And I would say, 'If I told you to stand up and show me your golf swing but you have to close your eyes, can you do that?' And they say, 'Of course,' and I ask, 'Why do you think that is?' and they say, 'I just know how to do it.'

You see, your muscles remember what you do, so if you've been practicing the golf swing, you've got the muscle memory of that golf swing.

What happens over time is if you use your muscles in a repetitive motion, the muscles remember. Then if you don't do yoga, or swim, or do something that's going to stretch your muscles out, over time your muscles will get shorter and shorter.

Then one day, you go to bend down and pick up the paper towel that fell on the floor, and all of a sudden you're grabbing your lower back and screaming, 'Oh my gosh, what did I do? My back just went out.'

Actually, that muscle got so tight, it formed a trigger point--a hyper-irritable spot in the muscle--and here's how trigger points work: If I pressed on your abdomen and pressed on that trigger point, you would feel it refer pain to the low back.

So a trigger point is kind of like a gun. You pull the trigger and it sends the bullet 200 yards straight out in front. When you have a trigger point, it's actually causing the pain to be referred somewhere else.

You see, your muscles remember where you put them...or what you do with them all the time, as in repetitive motions. So, if you go out and practice a golf swing, you're going to create new muscle memory with that new swing that you are practicing. Your body WILL remember that!

What happens over time is that we continually use our muscles in the same way over and over again. The muscles keep that memory and can eventually shorten (if they aren't stretched regularly) and will cause pain. A trigger point pain pattern can occur.

So, it's important to stretch these muscles when a patient comes in and re-educate the muscles to be longer...not shorter. Short, tightened muscles with trigger points cause up to 92% of chronic pain in the US!

Stretching is very important, and they also have to be the correct stretches. There are too many incorrect stretches being given to folks for their back pain. We'll go over that later...

Here's an example:

People rub their forehead when they have a headache but actually most headaches are coming from the side of the neck--the SCM (sternocleidomastoid) muscle--or the trapezius muscles on the tops of their shoulders. It feels good to rub your forehead when it hurts but that's not where the pain is coming from so rubbing your forehead won't make it go away.

It feels good to put ice on your low back when you have back pain but if you actually put a heating pad on the front of your tummy it would help much more, because that's the muscle that's tightened and shortened.

Kathryn: So where you feel the pain isn't necessarily where the problem is?

Frank: Exactly. I think the statistic is that 78% of the time the problem is not where you think it is.

If you're hurting in your knee, your knee is usually not the problem. It's not the knee so much as the rectus femoris, which is the main muscle that causes knee pain. It's one of the the quadriceps muscles in the front of the thigh.

Your knee pain could be coming from a trigger point up closer to the hip, believe it or not.

Kathryn: Okay, people get trigger points in unhappy muscles that get crabby, and then they go to the doctor and the doctor says…

Frank: He'll give them a muscle relaxer. He'll give them a pain pill. He'll say bed rest and, usually, when you rest in bed that might help but it's a temporary fix. Muscle relaxers really don't relax the muscles; they just make you kind of lethargic and you don't want to do anything. It makes you sleepy so in a way the muscles are resting but not truly.

Remember muscle memory? You haven't taken that muscle memory out of there. It's still tight, so when somebody comes into my office, I will find the why of their pain first. And then I don't just work on them but I educate them about how they can stretch that specific muscle that's causing the problem.

I help them learn how to get that muscle back to its full length. When the muscle is back to its full resting length, it stops causing pain.

The closer your muscle is to its normal resting length, the more strength you have in it. If a muscle's tight and shortened, it gets fatigued really quickly and can refer pain because it doesn't have any power to contract.

Kathryn: So the way you help people is by helping them figure out why they're having back pain or any pain?

Frank: Yes, and they like it because I tell them, 'I don't want to see you five times. I don't want to see you ten times. We want to find why you have it,' and I explain that to them in the consult.

Then I say, 'I want to educate you on how to keep this pain away because there's a reason you have this pain.' People like that because they feel empowered and they know that they have control now of what's been bothering them.

I can sometimes give a patient some suggestions over the phone once I have seen them so if they call up and say, 'Hey, I have something going on in my low back or up a little higher midway,' I might say, 'That might be this muscle, try this stretch.' So, I'll give them a stretch to do and typically they'll call me back a day later and say, 'Thank you so much, that really helped it and I feel better.'

I help them get the muscle back to its full normal functioning length. This brings it out of the pain range and the patient is very happy to have this happen.

So again, I'm giving them the power to get rid of this pain themselves and to help them figure out what caused it.

Kathryn: So when they go to the doctor, the doctor gives them some pain medication or a pill but you don't do that.

Why don't doctors do what you do? Why don't they treat patients as you do?

Frank: I think doctors have been trained to use medicine and that's what they do. I get to spend a lot of time with each patient. A doctor may have to see several patients in an hour.

I see seven to eight patients a day because I spend an hour with most patients. That gives me time to sit down and explain things to them and hear what's going on in their lives. Typically, I will hear patients, as they're telling these things, say, 'I've never had anybody ask me what I do during the day.' But, these things can be contributing to their pain.

And beside just the questions that I ask, they feel good about knowing they're talking to somebody who is really listening. They're letting out their feelings.

They're able to tell me, 'Oh that's right; the other day I did twenty bags of mulch and I was bent over a lot.' That helps them realize what contributed to their low back pain because they were shortening the front muscles.

Dr. Travell would say, 'The more you get a patient to talk, the more they're going to reveal to you.' This sure enough is true because I'll be talking as I'm working on a patient and they'll say, 'Oh, I forgot. I was walking out to the garage and I slipped on something. I didn't fall but I had to grab the bookshelf that was there and I really felt something grab right here.'

And, sometimes just that, a near fall where you save yourself, can be more traumatic than an actual fall because you engage so many more muscles when you're trying to prevent yourself from hurting yourself.

Kathryn: Why don't doctors have this information?

Frank: Think about it: Doctors have to know so much about the human body. That's why they have specialists for different fields. No one can know everything.

These last few years I'm getting more and more referrals from doctors who are aware of this kind of treatment. It's great that the word is getting out there.

I am trained in muscle pain and dysfunction. I believe doctors know a lot of things about our bodies but most aren't trained specifically in muscle function and pain just as I'm not trained as they are. That is why I'm writing this book. I want to help spread the word so more people can get rid of their pain.

I believe that one of the reasons doctors are becoming more aware of this treatment is because there are many more patients searching to find out why they are in pain and who want to get rid of it naturally. They don't want to be on pain pills. They don't want to be 40-years-old and not have a normal life anymore. This gets back to the doctors when the patients ask questions or when the patient lets them know that this therapy is what helped them.

We need doctors to help us and there are a lot of great doctors out there. I believe they have their hands full with all the illnesses and pain in this world. But no one can know everything about the human body and that's where someone with training like me comes in.

In fact, I often ask my patients to have a doctor look at their painful area first to make sure there's nothing real serious going on. Then I know it's safe for me to use my myofascial skills to help them after they have been cleared by the doctor.

More people than ever don't want to be on medication over extended periods of time. They would like to get back to a normal life and be pain free. That can happen. That's why you should never give up when trying to find the "why" of your pain.

It took me over 20 years to find the "why" of my own pain. BUT I DID!!!

We--you--should never stop trying to find the "why" of our pain. We all need to work together to eliminate chronic pain. Hopefully, we can all work together to achieve that common goal.

Many of my patients tell me that doctors are so busy right now that they can spend just a few minutes with you. Then they have to punch your info into the computer and say, 'Here are the medications.'

And, that's another thing, Kathryn!

Medications

The medications! Sometimes I ask my patients to bring in a list, actually all the time, especially if they're on a lot of medications because I want to see what they're on. You can have contra-indications to treatment or problems with mixing medications.

Sometimes there're two doctors involved and the doctors aren't aware of what the other doctor's doing.

I've had situations where I had to tell my patients, 'You need to go check this out and I'll look it up on the Internet and get a printout of the problems with the different drugs interacting.' And they're amazed that some medications or mixes of medications can be contributing to their pain.

Kathryn: And do some medications actually cause muscle pain themselves?

Frank: Oh yeah, sometimes the side effects are unbelievable.

I just saw a gentleman the other day who was having a problem and who was on one certain medication. I happened to have my iPhone with me and I punched in the medication and I said, 'So you're feeling lightheadedness, dizziness, and a few other things,' and he said, 'Exactly!'

Then I asked, 'When did this start?' And he said, 'Probably a month ago when I got on the medication.' I said, 'You need to talk to your doctor; look at these side effects.' And he was like, 'Oh, my gosh,' and he wouldn't have known to think about that otherwise.

So I sent him on his way and he's going to do well, I can tell.

Because we found the why.

Kathryn: You found the why.

Is surgery better for back pain than the therapy that you do?

Frank: You know, I had surgery on a shoulder one time because I had torn a muscle. I needed surgery but I first tried therapy, to see if that would take care of it, because I would much rather have someone try to release the muscles and work with me that way. I wanted to see if I could get my range of motion back with conservative treatment as opposed to surgery. I was still in pain after the trigger point treatment (two sessions.) That told me that something else was going on. Turns out I did need the surgery and I proceeded to get it fixed.

Each patient is different and has to be looked at carefully. There's no blanket statement to fit everyone. We can all have trigger points but WHY did we get them? The reason can vary from patient to patient.

With surgery, depending on what procedure you are having--shoulder, hip, leg or knee--you're out of commission for a few months easily while you recuperate.

If you get an MRI and you've seen tests that show you have a tear in the muscle, then possibly that needs to be repaired. But, many times they do not find anything. I often see this with patients who bring me their MRI reports. I will read the report and at the bottom of it is the impression of the doctor and there's nothing there about a torn muscle. Okay, so if the muscle's not torn, then I know there's a good chance I can help them.

Frozen shoulder: That's another thing people will have surgery for.

But why is the shoulder frozen? Because the muscles are tight. Something has somehow caused those muscles to get tight. Instead of surgery to release that shoulder, I can give you stretches to do, as well as work on you, and you can quite possibly regain most of your range of motion.

As long as there's no serious damage to the muscle or other soft tissues, trigger point therapy should generally work to regain what you've lost as far as mobility.

When the muscles are re-educated and back to their normal resting length, they won't refer pain into the lower back (or elsewhere) anymore.

Kathryn: Now what about physical therapy? Is it just as good as what you do? Is it different? How is it different?

Frank: Well, let's talk a little bit about physical therapy. I have had folks tell me that physical therapy was great and it worked for them. I also have had folks tell me it didn't work for them.

One thing is for sure, one modality or type of therapy can't fix everything and I get that. I don't think there's anything wrong with trying physical therapy if your doctor prescribes it. IF it doesn't work and or causes you more discomfort, then I think you need to try a different approach.

One place where we differ is that ice is used sometimes in their treatments. I, on the other hand, will never use ice on a muscle at my office. In my opinion, if ice is put on an area after it's been worked on this will contract the muscle and make it tight and short again.

I try to help my patients understand the difference between heat and ice so they know what to use and when.

Also, there are physical therapists who take this same training to give them another tool in their tool belt, so to speak, when they work with patients.

From my understanding, typically, physical therapists will try to strengthen the muscle. They feel a weak muscle needs to be strengthened but when you start contracting a weak muscle or a tight muscle, generally speaking, it is just going to make it worse.

When I see my new patients, they've typically been to physical therapy two or three times, or gone to two or three different physical therapists, and they say, 'It only hurt.'

And a lot of times, once they've worked on a patient, and this varies from physical therapist to physical therapist, they'll put ice on an area after they've worked on it. Now to me, ice is going to make the muscle contract and make it shortened again. I talked some about ice earlier.

Here's how I can help you understand the difference between heat and ice. Let's say I go out to get the newspaper and it's a nice summer day and I'm just in a pair of running shorts and my t-shirt. I can walk outside and I just stretch and say, 'It's so beautiful,' and I just absorb the warmth and the sunlight.

But, in February, if I go out in those running shorts and that shirt and I go to grab the newspaper, what do I do? I bunch my arms up together and I'm saying, 'Oh, my gosh, it's so cold!' So that's what your muscles are doing when you put ice on them for an extended period of time. The muscles just shorten up.

You want your muscles to be relaxed.

I don't want to add any contraction or any tightness or tension to those muscles especially after working on them. I'm going to put heat on them and let the heat help the muscles relax and those are some of the differences with physical therapy.

There are some physical therapists who do use Dr. Travell's protocol in their practices. I'm glad to see that more therapists are open to new ideas and can incorporate them into their practices just as I'm always searching for something that will and can help my patients.

So, the bottom line is, yes, there are differences between us, but we both help our patients. If I can't help my patient I then try and help them find "why" their problem is still there. It truly does take a village sometimes to help someone as opposed to just one person. While we may differ in our approach, we both do help people. The main point here is that we want to help our patients get well. We should listen to what the patient is saying and work from there with them.

Kathryn: You mean before the trigger points are relaxed.

Frank: Yes, you have to find why the muscle is tight and that's not usually addressed. It's not really addressed at too many places.

Kathryn: So when people have low back pain for one reason or another, they've done something or they slept wrong…

Frank: Or, they could've sat at a desk all their lives so they have muscles in a shortened position caused by sitting.

Kathryn: Okay. Or, they have the wrong kind of shoes or they have a Morton's Toe or their diet is doing something to cause their back pain.

Frank: Yes, ma'am.

Kathryn: What can they do to help themselves get rid of their low back pain?

Frank: Well, the first thing I do when they are in the office is give them the knowledge to know WHY they're hurting.

I give them the knowledge so they understand. I'll show them how to sleep. I usually also have them bring in pictures of what they look like sitting at home on the computer or in a recliner--which is not the thing to sit in because that shortens all the muscles that play into back pain--and I look at their postural pictures.

When I look at pictures of their sleep position they do not have to be asleep. They can be dressed in their everyday clothes. I have them lay on top of the covers with their pillow because I want to see how they position themselves at night.

Once I show them how to unwind, because they've been sleeping in a fetal position or really curled up, they're able to see that they can help themselves and they really do start to notice a difference within a day or so.

Sometimes, right after walking out of the office with the heel lift in their shoe and the correction in the shoe for the Morton's Toe, they can already sense that they are changing and that it's for the good.

When you're showing them why they hurt, that's what they want to know. Now they can say, 'Oh, okay, this isn't a mystery. I get this. Now I know why I am hurting,' and they feel they can combat it now.

It's not usually something that's going to be happening for the rest of their lives. I really try to let my patients have the power to help themselves and the knowledge of how to do it.

I'm always talking to them and I'm always educating them about why they're hurting. Often they'll have questions for me to answer when I'm working on them.

Kathryn: You just mentioned a heel lift. Tell us about the heel lift.

Frank: There are two important things I do when somebody comes in. I look at how they sit and I will give them an ischial lift to put under their sit bone if they need it. I can tell if they need it by the way they lean to one side or shift around uncomfortably. I also look at how they stand and I will give them a heel lift if they need one.

Whether we're sitting or standing our hips are engaged and, if you're uneven, it's going to make your muscles work against each other as opposed to working with each other.

Case in point: People who come in with fibromyalgia will say, 'I'm so wiped out by 2 o'clock. I'm just totally wiped out.' But, if they needed the heel lift and the ischial lift, they notice a difference in their stamina because all of a sudden, they're not using all their energy to try to right themselves all the time.

They're not leaning to one side and struggling to stand up straight anymore.

Their muscles are relaxed and they're not straining to try and keep their head level and things like that. The heel lift is a big deal because if you have one leg just a little bit shorter than the other, as many of us do, you're coming down on one leg harder than the other.

I've had patients come in complaining of knee pain. I will check to see if one leg is shorter (the hip height is lower.) If so, I then use a lift on the shorter side. I also check to see if they have Morton's toe. These two corrections can make a huge difference in how they feel.

I've had people with knee pain and the knee pain is gone, as a matter of fact, once the heel lift is in their shoe. Now they're able to tell that they're walking correctly and that their weight has been distributed properly.

To get the point of a heel lift across, I will tell them:

'I want you to think about the heel lift as a front end alignment. Think of it this way: You've got two tires on the front of the car. You've got a tire that is 15 inches wide on one foot and, on the other foot, you've got a 14 inch wide tire, so that's the shorter leg. And if you have an imbalance like that you're going to be pulling to one side if you're driving a car. That also goes for when you're standing and walking.'

You can sometimes see people with one hip that just really dips down when they walk because that leg is shorter than the other. Then we put that heel lift in there and, just as when a car has both tires the same size the car will run straight and true, so with the human body.

So there's a lot that goes on with the feet that affects posture and causes pain.

When you make corrections for Morton's toe and for the leg length differences with a heel lift, it changes people's lives. Their body senses it and they can see that they're going to perform better and start to live better.

Kathryn: So people have foot problems and that causes back problems.

Frank: Oh sure. I mean, think about the time that maybe you twisted your ankle and all of a sudden you're limping. You're trying to favor that ankle. Well, if you're doing that for a few days or a week, the limping movement is going to travel up your body into the hip and into the shoulder.

Anytime I see somebody who's wearing an orthopedic boot--if they've had surgery or maybe they sprained their ankle real badly—well, that boot is a lot thicker than your normal shoe. So, if somebody comes in and sees me I will tell them, 'You need that heel lift on the other foot, the good foot, to bring it even with the boot. That way, you're not going to throw off your hips and cause back pain or hip pain which can even affect your shoulders and your head.'

You need to have, at all times, your hips leveled.

I wear a lift in my right shoe and if I don't have it in there, within an hour or two, I can sense something is off. I start to get sciatic pain because I'm putting too much stress on the small muscle on the hip side, the gluteus minimus, which refers sciatic pain.

It's important to have everything balanced. That way your body's going to perform and function better.

That's what I help people do.

Chronic Pain: Sleep Position 101

http://budurl.com/Frank11

I made this video so you can see what the correct postures look like to sleep on your back. When your pillow is too high as demonstrated in this video, you are putting your muscles in a shortened position that will/can cause pain in the morning. You will have headaches as well as back pain. By having a pillow that is too high you are shortening the upper stomach muscles, chest muscles and neck muscles.

When the FRONT of your body is tight it will shorten the muscles in the front of your body and can contribute to your back pain. If you sleep with too many pillows (which raise your head too high) try sleeping in a nice, more neutral position as I demonstrate in this video.

A Good Side-Sleep Position

http://budurl.com/Frank12

Once I completed the first video on proper back sleeping I received a lot of emails asking for the proper side sleeping position. So here it is.

This position is usually a huge factor in getting folks to feel better when they have chronic back pain. I would say that sleep position and Morton's Toe play into back pain much more than most doctors realize. There's a video about Morton's Toe later. It's very important to sleep in a nice, neutral position so that your muscles are relaxed at the end of a nights' rest.

Too often folks have one leg rolled in front of the other which is twisting most of the stomach muscles and actually the whole lower back, too. You MUST sleep as demonstrated in this video so that most of the muscles are in a nice relaxed position and they won't be tight in the morning.

Think about it. We try to sleep for 6 to 8 hours a night. So, for 6 to 8 hours you are keeping those muscles contracted which are causing the pain that you have. Take a look and see how I used to sleep. It's no wonder that I had chronic pain for those 20 years!

Now, I'm pain free because of making these and other changes.

Honestly, it will take a few nights to get this correction down--but remember--you are teaching your muscles a new memory. Don't give up or get discouraged. It's like learning a new golf swing. You have to practice that new swing so that your muscles REMEMBER where to be.

Perpetuating Factors—How They Cause Your Pain

http://budurl.com/Frank13

This is a video on perpetuating factors--"things that cause your pain." I will go over a few things that you can change to make yourself better.

I would recommend the other videos on my YouTube channel as well so that you can get more information to help yourself. My YouTube channel is Paininvirginia. There should always be a "why" to your hurt. See if some of these sound familiar to you.

One Leg Longer Than The Other? Why Is That Important?

http://budurl.com/Frank14

If one of your legs is longer than the other it can, and will, throw off your hips and make them uneven. It can cause pain in the low back and also sciatica. You have to have level hips so your body can function correctly and smoothly.

This is the very first thing I check when a new patient comes in. It can be life changing for those who suffer and they don't know why. Plus it's simple to do...no surgery....no pills...just a simple lift in one shoe.

Questions? Email me and I'll be happy to answer.

Remember, you can find all of my videos at my YouTube channel
http://YouTube.com/PainInVirginia

Frank is a Myofascial Trigger Point Therapist who has been helping people get out of pain for many years.

Here's his story:

"I spent twenty-five years in a painting and wallpapering business but I had always thought that I was supposed to be doing something in the health field.

I had chronic pain for twenty of the years, too. I finally went and saw a Trigger Point therapist and was blown away that it was that easy to "fix me." I was hooked on Trigger Point Therapy from that day forward.

I was blessed enough to study and work with an expert who knew about Dr. Travell's protocol and has passed it on to me. I learned about finding the "why" of someone's pain before I even worked on them. This led to folks getting well with something as simple as just a "heel lift" or changing their sleep position. Releasing the muscles is a no brainer after that. I know I was trained by the best. There is no doubt in my mind and I feel very, very blessed about that.

Honestly, I knew God had a plan for me with this.

- Frank Gresham, CMTPT

Frank Gresham is a Chronic Pain Specialist who specializes in Myofascial Trigger Point Therapy. Trigger Point Therapy is a modality about muscle pain and how it affects our bodies. Over 92% of chronic pain comes from tight, shortened muscles and Trigger Point Therapy can be the answer.

Frank has given relief to hundreds of people with pain all over the world. Frank's journey started with his own pain of migraines and back pain that he had for over 20 years.

Many, many pain pills and doctors later he found out about Dr.Janet Travell's research on myofascial pain. This was a new beginning for him. The light bulb went on immediately when her protocol was applied to his own pain.

Now he has been pain-free for over 10 years and he wants to pass this on to anyone who is in chronic pain.

Frank says:

One of my favorite quotes from Dr.Travell is, "If you keep the patient talking, you will find the "why" of their pain." To this day it still holds true. I hope to help you find the "why" of your pain.

Frank has traveled to Norway and throughout the United States assisting in teaching Dr. Travell's protocol for myofascial trigger point therapy.

He is a graduate of the American Institute of Myofascial Studies and is a member of the National Association of Myofascial Trigger Point Therapists, the American Academy of Pain Management, and the International Myopain Society. Frank was an intern at the Shaw Institute of Myofascial Pain Treatment. He is a Certified Manual Trigger Point Therapist with extensive training in methods of natural pain relief.

Frank works and lives in Northern Virginia. His practice, "The Chronic Pain Center," is located in Springfield, Virginia.

Frank's website: http://TheChronicPainCenter.com

Frank was humbled to receive this message from the social-business networking site LinkedIn in 2013:

"Frank, congratulations! You're one of the top 1% most endorsed in United States for Chronic Pain.

LinkedIn now has 200 million members. Thanks for playing a unique part in our community." ~ LinkedIn.com 2013

http://linkedin.com/in/frankgresham